The Ma

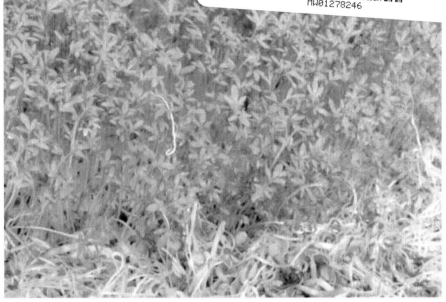

Natural Health Series

Dueep J. Singh

Mendon Cottage Books

JD-Biz Publishing

All Rights Reserved.

No part of this publication may be reproduced in any form or by any means, including scanning, photocopying, or otherwise without prior written permission from JD-Biz Corp Copyright © 2014

All Images Licensed by Fotolia and 123RF.

Disclaimer

The information is this book is provided for informational purposes only. It is not intended to be used and medical advice or a substitute for proper medical treatment by a qualified health care provider. The information is believed to be accurate as presented based on research by the author.

The contents have not been evaluated by the U.S. Food and Drug Administration or any other Government or Health Organization and the contents in this book are not to be used to treat cure or prevent disease.

The author or publisher is not responsible for the use or safety of any diet, procedure or treatment mentioned in this book. The author or publisher is not responsible for errors or omissions that may exist.

Warning

The Book is for informational purposes only and before taking on any diet, treatment or medical procedure, it is recommended to consult with your primary health care provider.

Check out some of the other Healthy Gardening Series books at Amazon.com

Gardening Series on Amazon

Check out some of the other Health Learning Series books at Amazon.com

Health Learning Series on Amazon

Table of Contents

Introduction

Nobody is quite certain when human beings decided to make sprouts a part of their daily diet. Not only were they healthy and nourishing, but they are also an unusual contrast to other vegetable and fruit items in matters of texture and flavor. But it is a well-known fact that millenniums ago, people of those cultured civilizations knew everything about adding germinating seeds to their daily diet, and did so regularly.

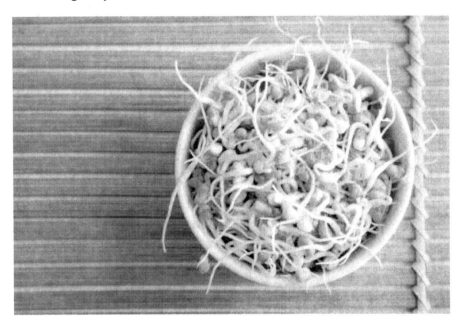

In olden days, people of many such civilizations worshiped the Gods and Goddesses of Harvest by offering them a handful of sprouted grains, before the first spring sowing of the year. So in one way they were appeasing the gods, and asking their blessings for a bountiful harvest. In another way, they were making sure that the seeds that they intended to sow in their lands were capable of producing plants through successful germination! So one could say that two birds were knocked out with just one stone.

Sprouting is the process of germination in which seeds, which are edible are allowed to grow into little plants. These are then eaten raw or they are cooked.

Sprouting is an integral part of East Asian cuisine, where traditionally nearly every meal had sprouts in some form or the other, either raw or in cooked form added to the platter. Luckily, this healthy habit spread throughout the world, and more and more people began to know all about the benefits of eating sprouts to gain nutrition and enjoy good health.

The Nutritive Value of Sprouts

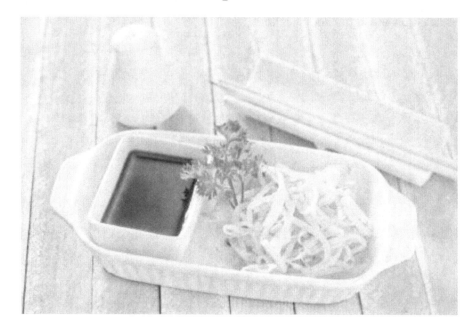

Even in olden times, people knew that sprouts had a very powerful nutritive base. That is why wheat sprouts were normally fed to expectant or lactating mothers, in many parts of Asia, so that their offspring were healthy. The minerals, vitamins, proteins and amino acids available in sprouts are easily digested. They are also necessary to keep you healthy

This germinating system is going to start as soon as you soaked dormant or resting seeds. The exposure to water breaks down complex compounds to make simpler compounds which facilitate germination. The seeds are also going to have vitamins A, B, C and E, amino acids, sugars and other essential nutrients in large quantities. There is an improvement of the quality of proteins in these seeds, thus making them beneficial for the health of those people consuming them in their germinated form.

Believe it or not, sprouts have vitamin contents which are **30 times higher** than those available in a mature plant. Mung sprouts have an increase of vitamin **B2 up to 515% during sprouting.**

Suitable Sprouting Seeds

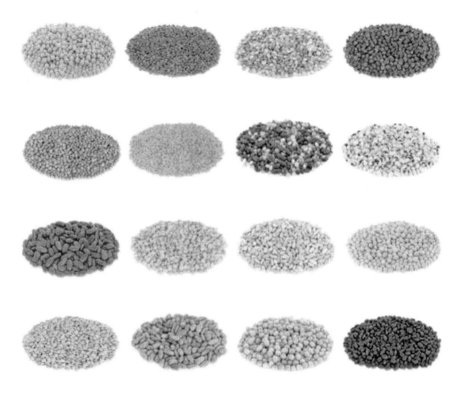

All edible seeds can be sprouted. But there are some sprouts, which are never eaten raw, but always eaten in their cooked form. There are also some plants whose sprouts are never consumed, because they cause health problems. These include plants of the Solanaceae family, which means you should not eat eggplant, potato, rhubarb or tomato sprouts. That is because the sprouts/seeds have toxic materials in them which are going to cause you digestive problems.

Also, there are those seed sprouts, which need a long time in cooking, especially beans. Their sprouts should never be eaten raw, but always cooked.

The suitable sprouting seeds from which you can grow sprouts are legumes and pulses and also plants belonging to the pea family. These include fenugreek, clover, lentils, peas, alfalfa, soybeans, and mung beans.

Mung beans are the most popular sprouted beans used for germination purposes all over the world.

The cereals which can be sprouted are corn, barley, oat, wheat, and rye. Amaranth and buckwheat are also pseudo-cereals, and their sprouts are also nutritious.

Oilseeds like hazelnut, sunflower, sesame, peanut, linseed and sunflower are also good sources of edible sprouts

The cabbage family, which includes turnips, cabbage, mustard, broccoli, radish, watercress, and other vegetable greens are going to provide you with good vegetable sprouts. Add them to your diet.

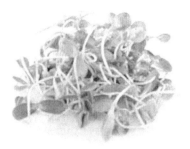 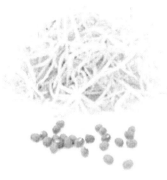

Herbs like onions, celery, parsley and fennel, especially those umbelliferous vegetables are good micro greens. So instead of using them as sprouts, use them as salads. Along with that, herbs and vegetables like lettuce, spinach, carrot and other such greens can be made into micro greens, which means that along with these grown vegetables harvested, you can even eat their small sprouted one-week-old plants, in the form of salads or just extra nutritious crunchies.

In Japan and in other parts of Asia the husk is removed before Rice is sprouted. The rice use here is brown rice. This rice is also excellent for sowing purposes.

For all those people who are interested in the best food with which they can reduce weight, as well as keep their hearts healthy, I would suggest Sprouts.

They are good for the heart as they are rich in fiber and natural antioxidants like vitamins C and vitamin E. Sprouts also help in reducing weight.

How to Use Sprouts

Sprouts can be eaten raw by the handful, or they can be stir fried in a Wok. You can also add them to salads, as a crunchy contrast to softer vegetables.

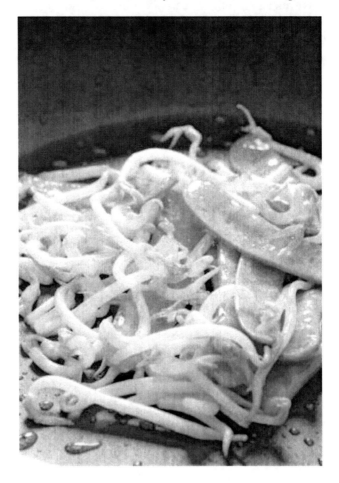

Sprouts can be easily germinated at home, even though they are being produced industrially and marketed all over the world. These marketed products are good options for those people who really do not have the time to sprout them at home, but according to Wikipedia, the FDA has begun to have a health concerns about bean sprouts made in contaminated soils, where they are infected by harmful bacteria and viruses.

Also, the consumption of raw sprouts very often is not advised, because there is always the chance of potentially harmful bacterial growth, especially if they have been grown in unhygienic localities and then packed for the global market.

Buying Sprouts

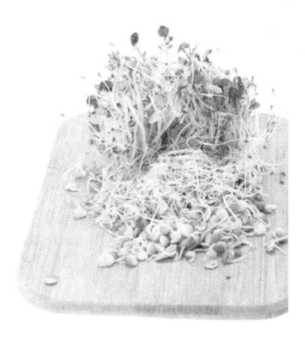

Even though I would suggest that you grow sprouts yourself at home, many consumers all over the world like to get their sprouts off the supermarket shelves. That is because sprouts are easily available at grocery stores, as well as health food stores.

The most popular sprouts available to you are radish sprouts, alfalfa, beans, sunflower, wheatgrass and of course mung beans

If you are buying them off the supermarket shelves, I would suggest looking at these particular tips and precautions

If you are buying them which have already been packaged, always turn over the container so that you can look at the bottom of the container. If it is damaged, that means the sprouts are definitely not to be eaten. The bottom of the container is going to show signs of spoilage and old age. This is going to affect the whole batch.

This is the reason why the FDA is so particular about sprouts, especially those coming from abroad, because there is always the fear of contamination and spoilage.

Sprouts are normally packaged in clear and small plastic boxes. They have drainage holes at the bottom which help the sprouts remain fresh.

I do not approve very much about buying anything, which has been packaged in a plastic bag, however much any department may tell me that that plastic is not harmful to human beings. I just do not like plastic. Nevertheless, most of the items which you buy in the market today are going to be packaged in plastic bags in case of spouts you have to be especially careful in checking them, because sprouts in plastic bags are going to spoil more easily. That is a proven fact restricted not only to sprouts, but also to mushrooms, and other vegetables like baby corn.

The roots of the sprouts should be green and they should smell fresh. The tops should have two tiny bright green leaves, if the sprouts are a bit older. If you are buying sprouts, which are micro greens, you may want to look at more greenery in the baby plant depending on your taste.

For the non-green bean type sprouts, look for a uniform whitish color and plumpness in the seedling from end to end.

If the rootlet portion and end of the sprout looks wilted, or the sprouts are tinged with any sort of brown discoloration, this means that they are old sprouts. They are going to be spoiled soon. So do not buy them.

The best sprouts are those which are crisp looking, plump and ones which look "alive! "

Radish sprouts and alfalfa sprouts grown in the half shaded sun are going to turn out a little bit green. That is because of the chlorophyll being added to them through the sun.

Make sure that you never pour hot water on the beans, while you are washing them before sprouting. This is the easiest way in which you can kill the germinating embryo.

If you happen to be traveling and are looking for healthy nutritious food, supplements, in order to keep you and your family healthy, look at the locally available seeds for sprouting. Avoid those seeds which you do not know, until you are back home!

If you are camping, make sure that the source of water with which you intend to irrigate the seeds is fresh. Do not use tap water if you are traveling in a country where you are not very familiar with the water sources used in the city.

Uncontaminated water is best, especially if you are hiking in federal parks or in state parks or in wilderness areas. Get that water straight from the water source.

Sprouts are excellent items to eat at Camp just like jerky and pemmican.

Why Are My Sprouts Inedible?

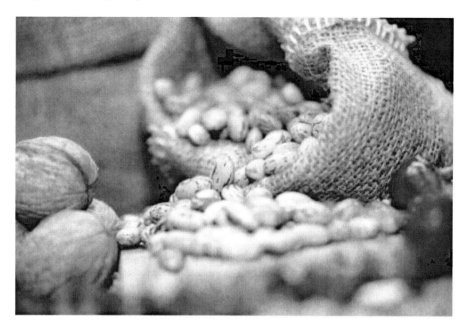

Seeds need moisture to sprout.

You may find your seedlings not growing sometimes. These are some factors which have caused your seedlings from failing to sprout.

If your seeds are allowed to dry, or are treated to eat, they are not going to germinate. They are not going to germinate in very high or very low temperatures. If you leave them to soak after you soaked them for a little while initially, – after rinsing – your seeds are going to catch "cold." The chances of their germination in such cases are thus considerably lowered.

Make sure that these seedlings are grown in areas where they can get some amount of sunlight. These seedlings are going to be much more nutritious. You can grow them in dark conditions, to get whiter and sprouts, which are crisp in texture, especially those which are so appreciated by hotels for cooking, but they are not so nutritious. So let them grow in the sun and add to their nutritive value.

Do not grow them in total sunlight. This is going to dry them out, because we have delicate seeds, which do not take well to overheating.

In China, traditionally a weight was placed on top of the seedling container. The result was crunchier and larger sprouts.

How to Make Sprouts

Sprouts can be made from any beans type and variety, even though lentils like mung are the most popular traditional mediums for making this nutritious addition to your diet. To make sprouts, you are going to dip a clean piece of cloth in water and then wring it out. Take your choice of grains/pulses and spread them all over that wet and moist cloth. Cover the grains with another layer of wet and moist cloth.

Keep for 36 – 48 hours, making sure that the water content on the cloth remains ever present because after all these seeds are germinating. After 48 hours, you are going to get sprouted grains, which can be eaten in the morning with breakfast, or whenever required.

Do not fry them in oil. If you are a heart patient, you may want to just dry stirfry in a wok and sprinkle it all over your food or add to your salad.

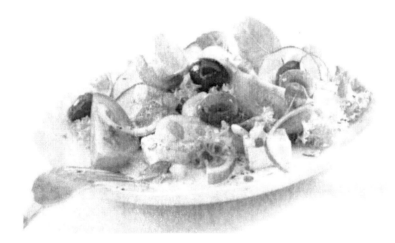

Try making salads a part of your daily diet. Sprouts can be added to these salads, and you can sprinkle some herbs on them to give them more taste and flavor. As you cannot use salad dressing because of the oil content, add some yogurt, which has been made by skimmed milk. Naturally, you would want to sprinkle some mung sprouts over them.

Yogurt is basically pasteurized or homogenized milk in which a bacterial culture has been added. This is a useful source of calcium and phosphorus. It also contains necessary vitamins like B 2 and B12, which helped to replace valuable bacteria in your digestive system and which also helps in the boosting of the immunity system.

Salads – with sprouts – can be taken throughout the day, and in whatever quantity you wish, as long as you do not smother them with mayonnaise or rich salad dressings. Just make sure that you are not underweight. If that is the case, you are going to tend to lose more weight. That is why salads are used for weight loss. That is because they provide a rich source of fiber and also provide more bulk to your diet. They also help eliminate the sugar and cholesterol present in your diet.

Cauliflowers and radishes included in your salads may produce flatulence. So add some fenugreek seeds or aniseeds to the salad.

https://www.youtube.com/watch?v=zk3jEE_8s1g is an excellent URL, where you can see how you can grow a varied and assorted mixture of sprouts. The beans you see in the video called peasant mixture include a number of beans and lentils like mung, garbanzo, red lentils, yellow lentils, chickpeas, etc.

I would suggest that you do the initial soaking in a colander. The maker of the video did the initial soaking in the jute bag itself. [You will learn how to make a jute bag further on.] That went to that all the dust particles remained in the jute bag. However, washing the beans in the colander is going to remove any vestiges of dust and pesticides.

Remember regular rinsing is necessary after every 12 hours to keep the beans well moisturized.

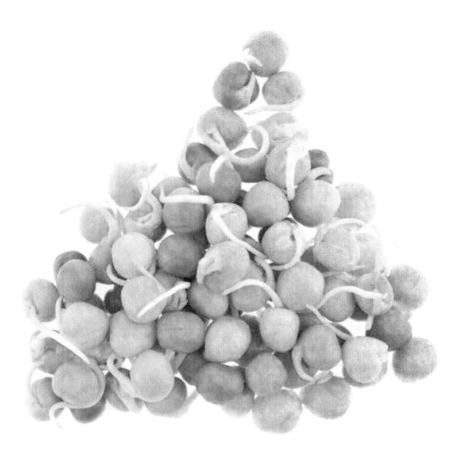

And as one watcher said in the comments column, do not use an aluminium utensil but use a glass container for washing. I say, use the colander. Do the initial soaking of the seeds in a glass utensil. In many parts of the East, earthenware cooking pots are still very much in use in the kitchen, that is why they are used for cooking and soaking purposes. So if you have them, so much the better.

Sprouting Lentils in Colanders

You may want to try out this method of sprouting lentils to be eaten in cooked or raw form, by just growing them in a colander.

You need to soak the lentils or the beans overnight in water so that they get ready for germination. Place them in a colander. Keep moistening them occasionally. The best thing about this growing method is that you do not have to bother about any sort of water stagnating around the seeds.

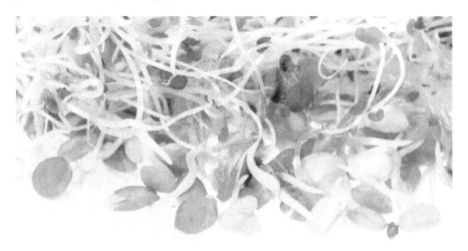

Making a Sprouting Bag

I was just moving around the local market, and I found that there were number of jute packaging sacks lying waste on the ground. Immediately something clicked in my mind and I thought to myself, "jute is the perfection material and natural fabric, which can be utilized effectively to make sprouting bags. That means one does not have to bother about moistened cloths to place on the sprouting seeds."

Jute is very popular in many parts of the world, to make articles of clothing, as well as sturdy bags, ropes, and other items of daily use. Hemp and jute are two different natural fibers altogether. Hemp is a natural fiber yielding crop supposedly seven – eight times stronger than another popular natural fiber yielding crop called cotton.

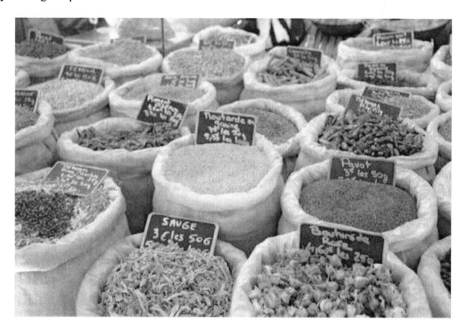

Herbs ,seeds and spices are traditionally stored in jute bags all over the world.

Jute is also a plant fiber, which is shiny and long. A number of these fibers are collected together and woven like one would weave cotton yarn.

So now I have a jute packaging sack in my hand. I need to make a bag, depending on the amount of sprouts, I want to grow.

Melissa has given excellent instructions on how to make a jute bag on this URL

http://www.ehow.com/how_8495877_make-jute-bags.html

I just cut the material from the sack, and sewed it together. My bag has a drawstring, instead of attached handles. This is so that I can make a bean sprout pouch

For that you need to Hem the upper edges of your bag. Measure off about 4 inches of the edge. Now, with the bag till turned inside out, turn the edges so that the hem allowance allows you plenty of space through which you are going to draw the drawstring. Use a very sturdy thread for hemming. Hem stitch all around the bag.

I found this URL so excellent, especially the explanation, so just make a sturdy hem.

https://www.youtube.com/watch?v=tMqK-fNrCrM

Then take a strong piece of string and thread it through your sprout bag. You need. You need not restrict your bag making expertise to just making sprout bags. Once you know how to make drawstring bags, you can make them whenever you have some spare material and some spare time going! They are always going to come in useful in the house to pack away the clutter.

Just place your seeds in the sprout bag

Readying Seeds for Germination

Make sure that the seeds are washed very well, so that any sort of remnants of pesticides are removed. Do not soak them in hot water, unless you intend to cook them instead of getting them to sprout.

Seeds are ready for germination when you look at them after an overnight soaking. They should be swollen up. They should also be plump in appearance. After that, rinse them once again.

A large percentage of my family members prefer to eat mung sprouts raw, especially when they are watching TV. They just sprinkle a little bit of their favorite herbal salt mixtures and a little bit of lemon on them and they are all set for a couple of hours of leisurely viewing. However, I like to cook my beans, after they have been sprouted. Remember that the more sprouted the beans are, the easier they are going to be to digest.

Cooked Beans, especially sprouted have a very unique and delicious taste. In fact, when I make my favorite beans, I know that is just soaking them overnight may not be enough in the digestion stakes. Besides, it takes so long to cook them. So I allow them to sprout for about 3 to 4 days before cooking them. So that does make an unusual bean curry, but I like this nutritious way of getting my beans along with lots of good taste and lots of good health.

How to Grow Wheatgrass Sprouts

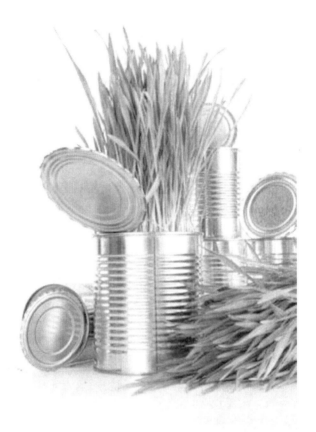

I know of an acquaintance who turned his terrace into a wheat crop growing farm, by just placing a waterproof tarpaulin over the cement surface, covering it with 8 inches of rich, loamy, organic soil and then sowing wheat on it. He harvested a bumper crop of rich golden wheat, which was the talk of the town. But you do not need to go to such drastic limits to get your crop of wheatgrass, especially when you are just making a couple of handful of wheat sprouts for daily consumption.

In fact, you can grow wheatgrass in boxes or even in large pots with a depth of about 4 inches and 1 ft.^{2} width.

If you are using wooden boxes or clay pots, baskets or big tins, you can fill them out with any type of earth as long as it is not sticky and Clay-ey. If you are in an area which is basically wheat growing, you can just go to a farmer friend and ask him for the best soil for growing wheat. You may want to borrow a sack full!

Make sure that the soil is free of chemical fertilizers. Natural organic manure is essential so that your wheatgrass grows in nutrient rich soil.

Do not buy chemical fertilizer – buy organic compost whenever you can, especially when you are buying something which is going to be used to provide nutrition for the grain you intend to eat.

Sprouting the Seeds Beforehand

100 grams of good quality wheat is going to provide you with 6 ounces of wheatgrass juice. This is enough for one day's quota for one healthy human being. Naturally, you are going to get hundred grams of sprouts too.

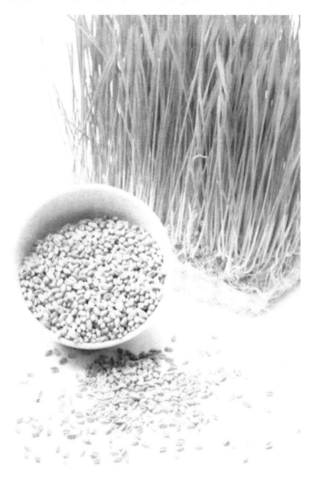

Before sowing the wheat, you need to sprout the seeds. That is done by soaking them in water for about 12 hours. Then wrap them up in a wet thick cloth and tie them tightly for another 14 hours. Keep sprinkling water occasionally on those sprouting seeds, to keep them moist.

As a result of this process, they are going to be sprouted well and you can see shoots appearing through the seeds.

This procedure of sprouting wheat prior to sowing is something quite useful, because you do not have to bother about the *will it sprout, will it not sprout* worry. This normally happens when the wheat has been recently harvested or may have been infested by insects and pests.

Thus, this pre-sprouting diminishes the chances of all your labor being wasted because the result after sowing and waiting eagerly for five days was a big lemon. Also, after soaking them in water and keeping them tightly wrapped, if only 50% of the wheat has sprouted, you can easily calculate that double the quantity of wheat is going to be required for sprouting and the subsequent sowing.

This will ensure proper statistics, quantities and an adequate yield in the necessary given time schedule.

Spread the sprouted wheat on the prepared soil bed in such a manner that the grains are close to each other and thickly sown. Cover them with a thin layer of soil.

Now sprinkle some water on these grains. Do not turn the hose pipe on them because overwatering is going to "spoil" those shoots.

Watering Wheatgrass sprouts/seedlings

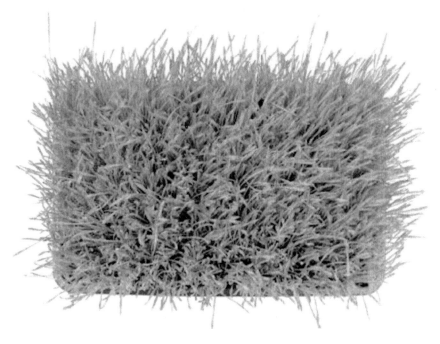

As wheatgrass grows really fast, you are going to get a good yield in around 4 to 5 days. The moment you see the seedlings sprouting, just water them once every 24 hours, but during the summertime, it may be necessary to sprinkle water on the seeds two – three times a day.

Watering the plants should be done either in the late afternoon or early evening.

The pots should be kept in the shade, especially in the afternoons. Do not expose those poor seedlings to the blazing hot sun.

Harvesting

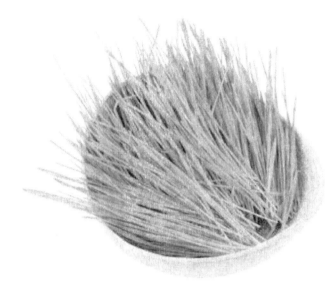

Do not allow the wheatgrass to grow more than 4 to 5 inches as the proportion of chlorophyll and other nutrients are going to start reducing from that time onwards.

Remember to do the sowing of the wheat every day for the initial six days so that you get a continuous supply throughout the year. So when you are ready to sow one lot, you are reaping another one.

Hundred grams are enough for one sowing. So by the time you have sown your last lot of hundred grams on Saturday, you have Monday's previously sown harvest ready.

Cut the grass with a pair of scissors as close to the bottom as possible. Watch it carefully to get rid of all the dust and the dirt. Put it in your blender and extract the juice from the grass. Never, ever pull the grass, up from the soil, as if you are de-weeding your crop.

After the grass has been cut, you can use the same earth again. But that needs to be spread and dried in the sun, and it is going to be ready for use after another three – four days. Add some more organic Fertilizer and rich loamy soil.

The temperature should be anywhere between 55 – 70°F or 13 – 21°C.

Any container which you are using to sprout seeds at home should have a good drainage system. That means that when you are going to moisten the seeds during the sprouting process, the water should not be allowed to stagnate on the surface. Any seeds that are sitting in stagnating water are not going to germinate. They are going to rot instead.

This moisture is going to cause the seeds to swell. Germination is going to start in 24 – 48 hours, depending on the seed variety, and temperature.

I was surprised to see that they are mung [by the way, the proper pronunciation of this particular bean is not mung, rhyming with hung, but *moong.*] sprout makers available in the market. Well, if somebody wants to spend some money, buying a utensil in which he is going to sprout beans, well, that is his outlook.

And also, because I am very budget conscious, and I am looking for the easiest way to use all my available resources to get the job done fast, you may want to look at this very interesting URL, with clear instructions on how traditionally, these mung beans were [and still are] sprouted in a container.

http://www.vegrecipesofindia.com/making-moong-mungsprouts-at-home/

Remember to rinse the sprouts a number of times a day, depending on the weather and the seed variety and type. This provides the seeds with moisture. It also prevents the seeds from souring.

The best harvesting time is when the seeds have been two – 3 inches in length. They are now suitable for consumption. If you leave them longer, they are going to develop and grow leaves. These are now known as micro-or baby greens.

The most popular salad baby greens are sunflower sprouts grown for about 10 days. If you want to halt the progress of growth of sprouts, just harvest them and put them in the refrigerator.

Mung Bean and Rice Pancakes

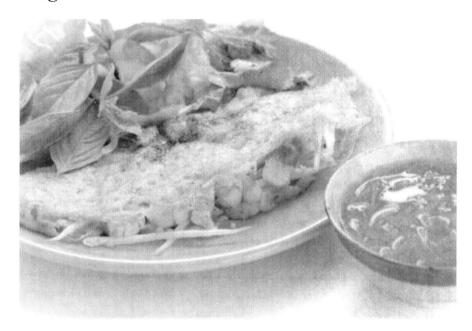

Banh Xeo- traditional mung – Rice pancakes. Delicious to look at, healthy to eat. Looks like they have been stuffed with shrimp, along with other herbs and greens.

The Vietnamese like a number of other ancient civilizations in the East love sauces with different tastes like sweet, sour, bitter, pungent, spicy or mild. That is why you are going to get alternating tastes and flavors in just one sauce like sugar, chilies, lime juice and soy.

So these pancakes are going to be accompanied with contrasting sauces with a sweet and sour flavor.

For the pancakes you need half a cup of long grain rice, half a cup of mung beans, three, thinly sliced onions, a pinch of turmeric, ¼ cup of coconut milk – this is traditionally an Eastern dish, that is why the onions and coconut as exotic ingredients – 2 cups of sliced mushrooms, 8 ounces of tofu or cream cheese drained and sliced into slices, a pinch of turmeric, 2 cups of mung bean sprouts, salt and pepper to taste, and the herbs of your choice like

mint, basil, thyme, cilantro or coriander for garnish and adding to the pancakes. 2 cups of a mixture of herbs is going to do very well.

Soak the rice and the mung beans overnight and separately after they have been washed and rinsed thoroughly. Drain the rice, wash again, and then grind to a smooth paste. Set apart.

Drain the beans and rinse them. Grind them into a paste. Add this paste to the rice paste mixture. Also add the salt, pepper, turmeric, chopped onions, and the coconut milk. Also add the chopped herbs as you prefer, leaving some for garnish purposes.

Now, heat some oil on medium heat in your griddle or on a skillet. Add the mushrooms and the tofu and stirfry until the mushrooms are just tender. I normally do all my stir frying in a Wok because the heat is so even.

Add just that amount of rice and mung batter to the vegetable mixture, so that the bottom of the pan is covered with a thin coating. Reduce this heat to low and cook until you have a crispy omelette like pancake.

Scatter some mung sprouts on one side of this pancake and fold like you would fold an omelette into a half pancake. You may want to turn the pancake Upside down without breaking, if you are a good cook and want the top portion cooked too, and browned. Each side takes about one – two minutes for cooking properly.

You can make six pancakes, with the tofu and vegetable fry mixed with rice and mung sprout batter. You serve these pancakes hot with spicy sauce. These pancakes are called Banh Xeo in Vietnamese.

Spicy sauce

This spicy sauce which is used for dipping the pancakes is a popular sauce which is normally used as a spring roll dip or a salad dressing. **For this you need one tablespoonful of lime juice and sugar and one teaspoonful of garlic and chili made into a paste. Along with that, you are going to add 2 teaspoonfuls of another sauce, which can also be used as a fish sauce.**

Mix all these ingredients together and use it as a dip for your pancakes.

Fish sauce.

The fish sauce is made by mixing ¼ cup each of brown sugar and soy sauce, 3 tablespoons full of lime juice and rice vinegar, one red ripe chili, chopped and four cloves of minced garlic. Add 5 tablespoons full of boiling hot water into the sugar. Mix until the sugar is dissolved. Allow to cool and then add the rest of the ingredients. Mix well. Refrigerate it. This is a fish sauce in which you can dip pieces of fish. You are going to use 2 teaspoonfuls of this particular fish sauce to make the spicy sauce for the pancakes.

Live Long and Prosper!

Author Bio

Dueep Jyot Singh is a Management and IT Professional who managed to gather Postgraduate qualifications in Management and English and Degrees in Science, French and Education while pursuing different enjoyable career options like being an hospital administrator, IT,SEO and HRD Database Manager/ trainer, movie , radio and TV scriptwriter, theatre artiste and public speaker, lecturer in French, Marketing and Advertising, ex-Editor of Hearts On Fire (now known as Solstice) Books Missouri USA, advice columnist and cartoonist, publisher and Aviation School trainer, ex- moderator on Medico.in, banker, student councilor ,travelogue writer … among other things!

One fine morning, she decided that she had enough of killing herself by Degrees and went back to her first love -- writing. It's more enjoyable! She already has 48 published academic and 14 fiction- in- different- genre books under her belt.

When she is not designing websites or making Graphic design illustrations for clients , she is browsing through old bookshops hunting for treasures, of which she has an enviable collection – including R.L. Stevenson, O.Henry, Dornford Yates, Maurice Walsh, De Maupassant, Victor Hugo, Sapper, C.N. Williamson, "Bartimeus" and the crown of her collection- Dickens "The Old Curiosity Shop," and so on… Just call her "Renaissance Woman") - collecting herbal remedies, acting like Universal Helping Hand/Agony Aunt, or escaping to her dear mountains for a bit of exploring, collecting herbs and plants and trekking.

Our books are available at
1. Amazon.com
2. Barnes and Noble
3. Itunes
4. Kobo
5. Smashwords
6. Google Play Books

Check out some of the other JD-Biz Publishing books
Gardening Series on Amazon

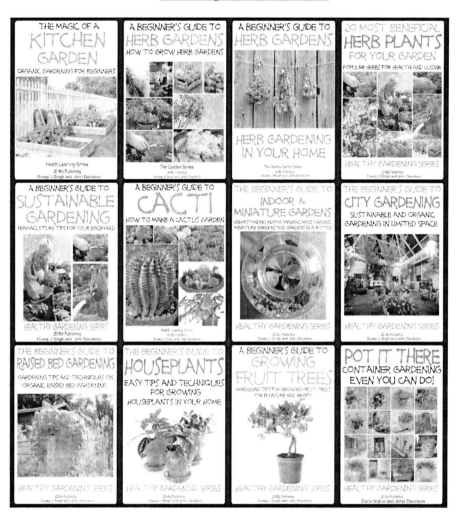

Health Learning Series

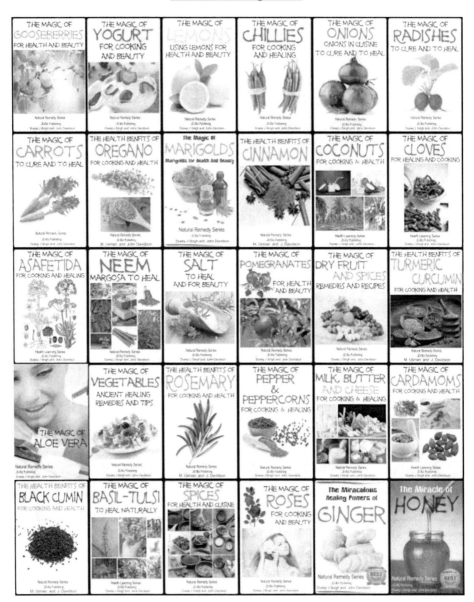

Country Life Books

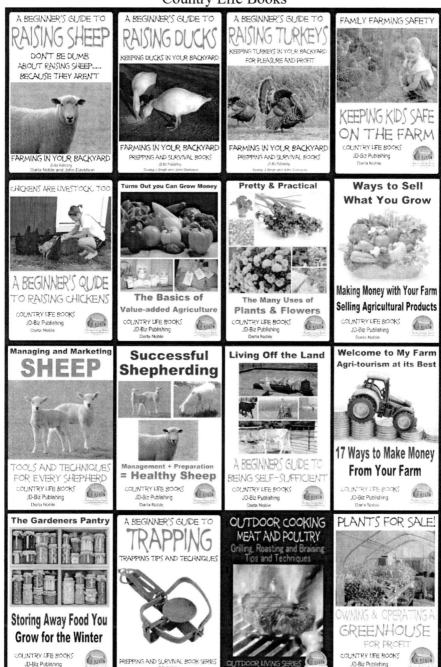

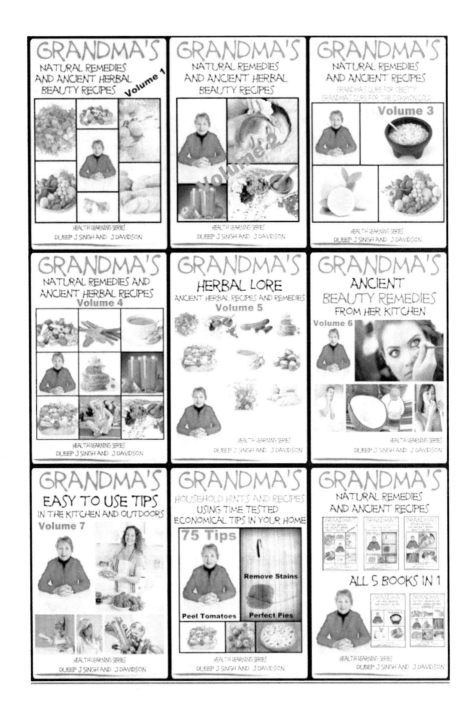

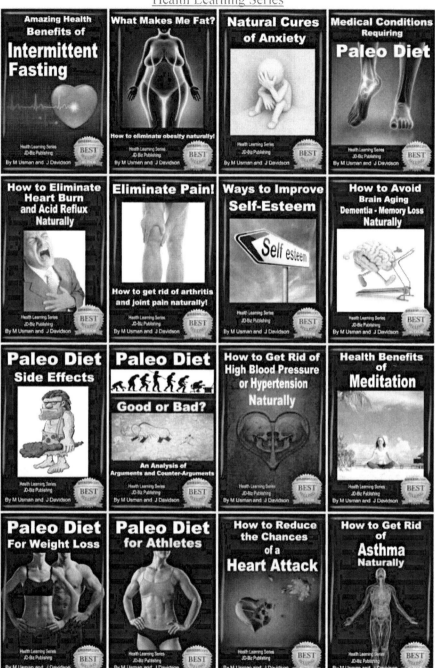

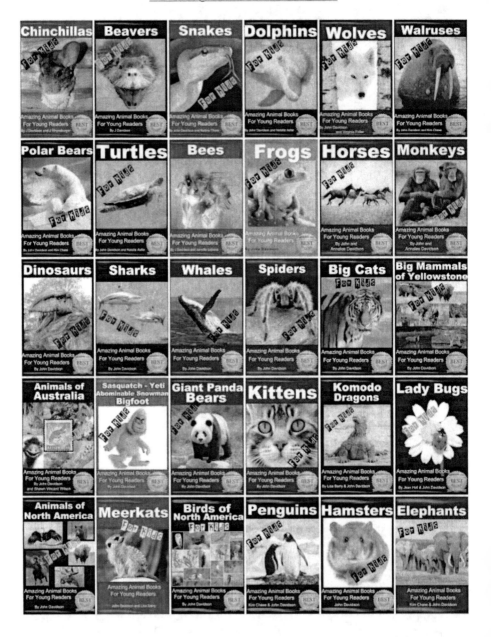

Learn To Draw Series

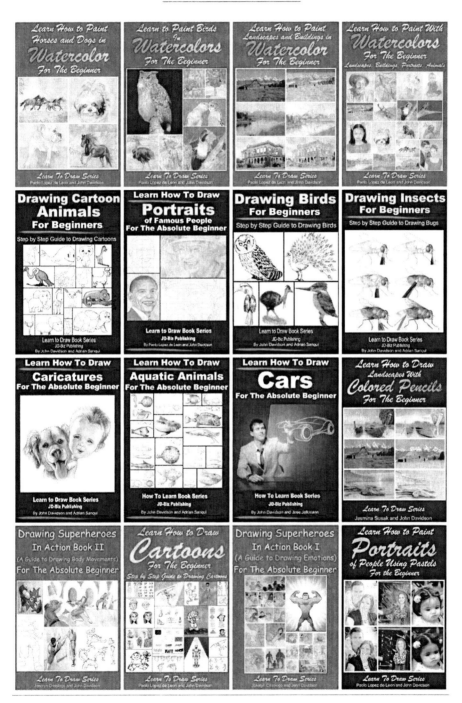

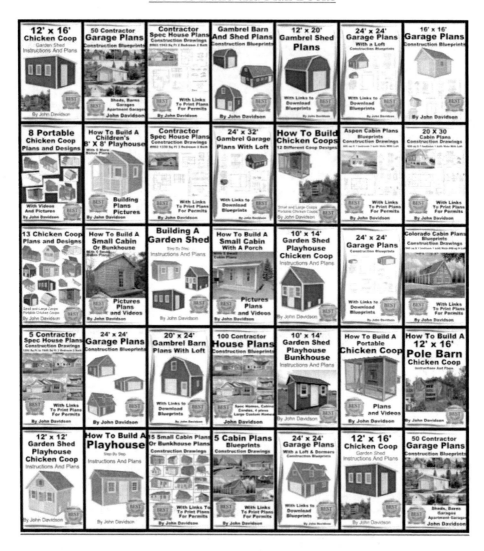

Entrepreneur Book Series

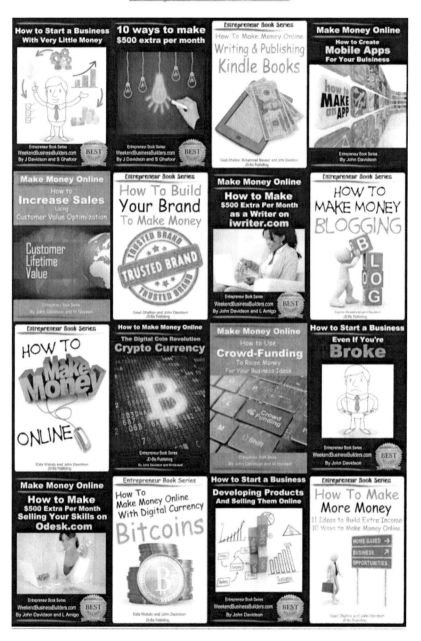

Publisher

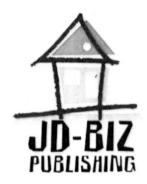

JD-Biz Corp

P O Box 374

Mendon, Utah 84325

http://www.jd-biz.com/

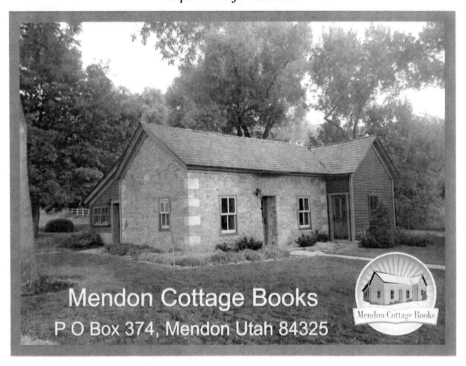

Mendon Cottage Books
P O Box 374, Mendon Utah 84325

CPSIA information can be obtained at www.ICGtesting.com
Printed in the USA
LVOW07s1640130116

470477LV00019B/1132/P

9 781505 631593